HOW TO LIVE VICTORIOUSLY EVERYDAY

BY.

TABOT HENRY OJONG

DEDICATION

- My profound and deep sense of gratitude goes to God Almighty who believes in me enough to commit the task of this book into my hands, and has helped me tremendously in every aspect to get the job done. Truly, we're nothing without God.

- This book is therefore dedicated to God Almightywho loves you and me so much that He wants nothing but the best for every one of us. And to all the people around the world who have almost given up on their dreams because of seeming defeat that stirs them in the face. I pray that these precious revelations will give you the strength you need to keep moving forward in destiny with giant strides. Peace!!

ACKNOWLEDGEME NT

- My thanks to the long list of spiritual fathers and authorities on this side of heaven whom God has raised for Himself, and whose insights and wisdom has enriched my life so much.

- For the endless love and support that my entire family and in-laws have given to me, words are not enough to express my gratitude. Even so, thank you. To the entire spiritual family and staff at Ever Winning Faith Mission you will always mean so much to me.

- To my biological children, I say, you'll always be my playmates and a key motivation to be a good role model.

- My Special thanks to my beloved wife, Charlotte, for her unconditional love for me, her commitment to the kids and the ministry; and her loyalty to our dreams and aspirations in life. To you, I say you will always be my soul mate and friend. I love you.

Table of Contents

INTRODUCTION

As it has been from ancient times and continues to be even today, many people wind up in the journey of life as failures and weaklings on daily basis because they came across mountains which they mistakenly interpreted as insurmountable - an ideology which left them completely overwhelmed and depleted of the vital energy needed to make forceful advancement in life.

Knowing the battles he would have to fight to conquer the promised land, God told **Joshua** this, no less than three times: ***"Be strong and of good courage."*** Anytime you move forward, obstacles will block your path. Count on it! **H.G. Wells** asked, ***"What on earth would a man do with himself, if something did not*** *stand on his way?"* what did he mean? He meant that adversity is your friend – even when it feels like your enemy. Every obstacle you face reveals your strengths and weaknesses. It also shapes and makes you wiser and more confident. **Poet Ralph Waldo Emerson** wrote: *"whatever you do, you need courage. Whatever course you decide upon, there is always someone to tell you that you are wrong. There are always difficulties arising*

That tempt you to believe your critics are right. To map out a course of action and follow it to an end requires some of the same courage that a soldier needs. Peace has its victories, but it takes brave men and women to win them." Anytime you leave your comfort zone and step out in faith to follow God, you will be tested. But you will also reach heights you thought were beyond you and go further than others who had greater talent but settled for the status quo. Friend, when it comes to everyday living, you can walk according to the unchanging principles of God's word or by your constantly changing feelings. When you live by God's word, you have stability. When you live by your feelings, it's like riding a roller coaster; one day you're up, the next day you're down. God wants to bring you into emotional maturity, but you have to cooperate with Him. This calls for a daily act of your will; choosing to do things His way rather than your own. And once it becomes a habit, you discover that life is more enjoyable. Now, you don't let everyone who knocks on your door come in and make themselves at home, so why would you let every emotion that surfaces dictate the direction of your day or decide your response?

Living by faith, as we know it, is something you learn to do by practicing it daily. Before you became a Christian, you trusted in your own ability and intellect. But those things only took you so far and no further, right? Now you're trusting God for the wisdom, guidance, resources, and ability to fulfill His will for your life. Faith doesn't stand to make things easy, faith only makes those things possible for you. Faith doesn't mean your problems will suddenly vanish into thin air, faith only gives you the assurance of victory no matter how controversial the evidence might seem. And that's why nine times out of ten, living by faith doesn't always make sense. Faith is a great catalyst for change – sometimes faith changes your circumstances; other times it changes your perspective. How? By giving you the tenacity to hang in there. When your bank balance shows a red signal, or the doctor's report is negative, or your marriage has turned into complete garbage, or the kids are running amok, or the company that has been your primary source of sustenance for the past 25 years suddenly winds up and closes its doors, faith gives you the fortitude to endure, confident that God will work things out on your behalf. As

Herbert Kaufman rightly said, *"The habit of persistence is the habit of victory."*

The mistake many of us make is always talking about what we intend to do tomorrow failing to realize that today is the tomorrow we talked about yesterday. In the midst of countless attacks coming at us on every side, what we need to do is redirect much of our energies and forces to bear on the present challenges to deal with them daily as they present themselves. We must learn to face life with one leg firmly planted in the present and the other seeking for a solid ground in the future. Focusing on the burden of the long distant future while neglecting the demands right in front of us is what has made countless multitudes to give up on their dreams in life before they even had the chance to start pursuing it or living their ideal life. And you know, Satan will try to discourage and defeat your aspirations by making you feel overwhelmed by the challenges. That's when you need to counter- punch, by breaking down your goals into smaller steps and live them out daily. **Abraham Lincoln** blessed my heart greatly when he said, ***"The best thing about the future is that it comes to us one day at a***

Victory and you can access that grace on daily basis.

This book will show you just how to press the

necessary power buttons that will keep you flying on

the path of victory every day.

CHAPTER ONE

YOU CAN LIVE VICTORIOUSLY AGAINST ALL ODD

If I shut up heaven that there be no rain, or if I command the locusts to devour the land, or if I send pestilence amongst my people; if my people, which are called by my name, shall humble themselves, and pray, and seek my face, and turn from their wicked ways; then will I hear from heaven, and will forgive their sin, and will heal their land. (2 Chronicles 7:13-14)

"There is a stranger in the house," my wife would normally say to me. ***"Very well then, prepare for him a delicious plate of rice and stew"*** I would normally respond. This way we jokingly communicate about the presence of a rat in our home and the need to get rid of it with some form of rat poison.

Shortly after my wife got delivered of our first child, she decided to pay a visit to her parents for a few weeks. Within that time, I got up one afternoon and went to the kitchen to fix up my lunch. As I entered the kitchen, I immediately noticed the presence of a rat running around and if there is one thing I hate to see in the house, it is a rat. There were these two 20-litres "panted" buckets standing on the floor that I saw it running over, so I decided to remove their lids and fill each with 10litres of water peradventure it comes out to run over them again and this time gets trapped due to the absence of the lids. With that, I walked out of the kitchen only to return forty minutes later and find it inside the water struggling for its dear life. I stood there for twenty more minutes and watched as the rat kept struggling to swim its way out. It kept pushing itself up even as the force of gravity kept pushing it to the bottom of the half-filled container. As I watched on, with folded arms I asked the rat, ***"Why are you struggling? If only you knew that there is no way out of the battle you*** *are in, and that I am the only one who can help you now, if I so choose to.* " Suddenly, the still small voice of the Holy Spirit came speaking to my heart *"much the same way many of you struggle with battles you just can't win on your own and end up dying when you could have called on me to help you out of your struggles.* " What a life changing revelation these words were to me!

Could that be a vivid picture or befitting description that suits you?

Reading this book right now? Have you unknowingly declared a

Downward spiral or doomed destiny for yourself by fighting on your own battles that you just can't win unless God helps you, but you just won't call on him? At the end of the twenty minutes I stood there thinking on what the Holy Spirit had just said to me, the rat ran out of strength, sank under the water and at that point, it was all over for the rat. Like this **_"smart but unfortunate"_** rat, I hope you don't end up dying in the devil's trap for you when you can simply call on God to fix things up for you. It is a fact that many people are sick and tired of their ugly situations in life, but it is even a greater truth that very few of these people are sick and tired of being sick and tired- these are the few who ever arise to do something about their situation, as we see in the following scripture.

But, brothers, when we were torn away from you for a short time (in person, not in thought), out of our intense longing we made every effort to see you. For we wanted to come to you – certainly I, Paul did, again and again – but Satan stopped us… so when we could stand it no longer, we thought it best to be left by ourselves.

(1 Thessalonians 2:17-18; 3:1, NIV)

From the passage above, we can see that Paul the Apostle had a mission to the brethren at Thessalonica but the mission was being frustrated because Satan did everything he could to stop their plans. When the Apostle Paul says, ***"we were torn away from you for a short time in person, not in thought"***, it implies the fact that their challenge was a reality, not some imaginary obstacle they were merely thinking might show up along the way. They were not merely trying to foresee what can possibly go wrong with their mission, he was talking about real problems they had in their hands when the Apostle also said, ***"For we wanted to come to you – certainly I, Paul, did, again and again,"*** what he meant was that he couldn't vouch for others how serious they were about the mission but he personally was, and that's why he was quick to pick out the fact that there was a resistance against their progress and he could tell where the resistance was coming from *"but Satan stopped us"*.

So when this Apostle on a mission became spiritually acquainted with the situation they were in, what did he do? Did he just fold his arms, sit by and accept Satan's verdict as final? No, I love what he did. He Reported.

So when we could stand it no longer, we thought it best to be left by ourselves in Athens. (1 Thessalonians 3:1, NIV)

Being left to themselves here do not imply a resignation to fate but a disposition of men who decided to take charge of their situation. They didn't just want to stay isolated from the crowd for nothing, they separated themselves so they could fully give themselves to the place of prayer as they sort to address the issue by the Spirit. Much like what the Apostles did when they had some problems to handle in the early church. *(Acts 6:1-4)* And what Jacob did when he needed some things in his personal life to turn around *(Genesis 32:1-28).*

When God deals with you on important issues, He does it one-on-one, not as part of the crowd. In fact, being in a crowd can keep you from hearing His voice. Being alone with God can feel threatening because your façade and ego gets stripped away. Your first impulse may be to stay with the crowd, but you soon discover they can't calm the restlessness in your spirit. That restlessness is God calling you to a

Meeting! So, like Jacob, don't be afraid to wrestle with Him until a new day breaks for you.

The principle and practice of being alone to sort things out with God is both an old and a New Testament concept as we can see from the passages above. If you must live this life victoriously at a very personal level in the midst of a failing multitude, then the practice of private prayer is unnegotiable for you. As Collins Brobbey rightly said, "If you want to be powerful, pray more privately and less publicly. But if you want to be popular, pray more publicly and less privately." Along the same line, Blaise Pascal also tried to shock the people of his days into seeing this. He wrote, "imagine a number of men in chains, all under the sentence of death, some of whom are butchered in sight of others; those remaining see their own condition in that of their fellows, and looking at each other with grief and despair await their turn. This is an image of the human condition." He was right especially when we consider the plain truth and harsh realities of human existence in this wild wicked world. But Mathew Henry was also right when he said, "When God intends great mercy for His people, the first thing He does

Is to set them a-praying."

True, Satan is on a mission to steal, kill and destroy amongst us. But don't forget that if the devil thinks he knows how to spoil things for us, our God much more knows how to fix them for us. If the promise in *2 chronicles 7:14* is true, and it is because all of God's promises are, then we can be confident that God has a good future for us, no matter how dark and sordid our past. Revival is what happens when spiritual vitality is restored to our hearts, as genuine prayer comes only from humble hearts. God demands for us to seek after Him but the truth remains that we can't seek God's face if we have been seeking something else. When a man gets to despair, he knows that all his thinking will never get him out, he will only get out by the sheer, creative effort of God. Consequently, praying puts him in the right attitude to receive from God that which he cannot gain for himself. Prayer therefore is a key element in walking the straight and narrow in a crooked world.

POSSESSING YOUR GLORIOUS DESTINY

It costs us nothing to walk by faith but it might cost us everything not to walk by faith. It is painful not to pray even more than it is to pray. It cost us only a little effort to pray but it might cost us our lives and

Destinies not to pray. The man who is not ready to pray is the man who is not willing to go far in life: And what's more? The people who don't look up to God always end up getting crowned with shame.

They looked unto him, and were lightened: and their faces were not ashamed.

(Psalms 34:5)

It is very easy to be disgraced with failure in life because it is the natural outcome of doing nothing worthwhile. What we always pray for is the grace of God to be released on us, never disgrace. Why then is it that so many professing Christians end up with disgraceful outcomes in life when they never prayed for it? It is because they didn't pray for grace either. I hope you are learning something here- that when you pray, grace comes and when we don't pray, disgrace is inevitable. Many men who have tried to continue the farce of rebellious independence from God are about to collapse because their strength has come to the end of the line. Everyone dumps their garbage on them, and they have no place to release it. Beneath the religious façade, many people are overwhelmed and stressed. They are secretly depressed and

Disenchanted. They have become their own god, so they must assume responsibility for the outcome of all issues. ***Reinhard Bonnke*** said ***"By our prayer, God brings things about that He would not do without prayer. It is not a matter of changing God's will but of praying that His will be done."*** God's will for you is success and the strongest force on earth that can bring that will into enforcement is the force of prayer.

A scientific law states that ***"Everything assumes a state of rest until a relevant force is applied to it."*** If you sit up, you will at once go up but if you sit still, your glorious destiny has no choice but to go stale. A man's obstacles only sit down when he rises up, and the world will only stand up for the man who will not sit down. The door to failure is wide open before every one of us. It is the door to success that we need to force open. It takes little errors to fail but it takes much efforts to succeed. Success will demand more from you in a year than failure ever will in a lifetime. Most important to note here however is the fact that failure will only continue in your life for as long as you continue to permit it.

WHERE THERE SEEMS TO BE NO WAY

You cannot overestimate the power of prayer. Prayer is as vast as God because He is behind it. Prayer is as mighty as God because He has committed Himself to answering it. If only you can bring yourself to the altar of prayer, God says;

Call unto me, and I will answer thee, and shew thee great and mighty things, which thou knows not. (Jeremiah 33:3)

Behold, I will do a new thing; now it shall spring forth; shall ye not it? I will even make a way in the wilderness, and rivers in the desert.

(Isaiah 43:19)

Prayer is the only guaranteed way out you and I have.

Prayer is all we can do because all we have is God.

That's why when you don't pray, God sees you as a

proud person-someone who says I can do it on my

own. Any morning you get up from bed and refuse to

pray, you indirectly say to God **"I don't need you."** If

you live a prayerless life altogether, then you have

indirectly but boldly declared to God **"I don't need you

in my life."** No doubt many people keep struggling

with

Failure all their lives? Failure in prayer is failure in all things. Planning to succeed in life without praying is playing without knowing. If you think you can manufacture your own way out, hear this;

DO YOUR DESTINY A FAVOUR

But we will give ourselves continually to prayers, and to the ministry of the word.

(A

The trouble with our praying is we just do it as a means of last resort. I may not know you personally and I may not know how much value you attach to prayer but I must state, sincere prayer is the heart of a happy and productive life. Prayer strengthens faith. Prayer is the preparation for miracles because when God steps in, miracles are bound to begin, just as our confusion is

bound to come to an end.

And though the Lord give you the bread of adversity, and the water of affliction, yet shall not thy teachers be removed into a corner anymore, but thine eyes shall see thy teachers: And thine ears shall hear a word behind thee, saying, this is the way, walk ye in it….(Isaiah 30:20-21)

Prayer then should be a lifestyle to help us maintain fellowship and promote or enhance our connectivity with God. You pray in your distress and in your need; would that you might also pray in the fullness of your joy and in your days of abundance. What a service you will do to your life and destiny if you don't allow your prayers to begin when all your other options run out, as in, ***"All we can do now is pray"*** No, other options can come and go but prayer would remain. Prayer is not merely an occasional impulse to which we respond when we are in trouble. Prayer is and should be our life attitude. God is not a cosmic bell-boy for whom we can press a button to get things. I think any prayer on our part should be a conscious response to what God is already doing in our lives, not merely what we hope and expect he will do.

There is need for prayers to go on always in our homes. A family that prays together stays together. Let prayer altar be raised here and there and let the prayers be loud, proud and unapologetic. To be a Christian without prayer is no more possible than to be alive without breathing. As a Christian, one question I want to ask you is this: ***"Is prayer your steering wheel or your spare tire?"*** if prayer were to be a talent then I would proudly say that the greatest and best talent that God gives to any man or woman in this world is the talent of prayer. But the truth is- Nobody has the gift of prayer. There is no such gift in existence. Whatever level of prayer a man now operates in, he grew to it through continuous prayer and constant repetition.

If we don't learn to kneel in prayer, we will stand in frustration. Our angry ranting and raving is only a telltale sign of how long it has been since we had fervent prayer! ***E.M. Bounds*** said that ***"Prayer is the language of a man burdened with a sense of need."*** When a man is at his wits end, it is not a cowardly thing to pray; it is the only way he can get in touch with reality. God is waiting eagerly to respond with new strength to each little act of self-control, small disciplines of prayer,

Feeble searching after him. And His children shall be filled if they will only hunger and thirst after what he offers.

A WORD FOR YOU

"Until you know that life is war, you cannot know what prayer is for"

-Daniel Henderson.

CHAPTER TWO

WHAT YOUR PRAYERS CAN DO

Whatever prayer or supplication is made by any or all of your people Israel-each man knowing the affliction of his own heart, and spreading forth his hands towards this house (and its pledge of your presence)- Then hear in heaven, your dwelling place, and forgive and act and give to every man according to his ways, whose heart you know, for you and you only know the hearts of all the children of men, that they may fear and revere You all days that they live…(1 Kings 8:38-40, Amp)

The bible is such a compact disc of instructions and revelations meant to do us a lot of good in the journey of destiny. Often times, it happens to be more demanding on us than any of us would love it to be. But reading from the above passage, we come across a very powerful and interesting prayer coming from someone who had experienced the many sided challenges of life and has encountered God in the process of rising to the top of the success ladder. As a man with large heart full of understanding and compassion for the struggles people go through to earn a decent living, *King Solomon* prayed and asked God to release divine assistance to those who attach importance to it, to those who are sick and tired of laboring into emptiness and to all those who are humble enough to seek the face of God over their particular situations. I love the particular line in his prayer that says ***"Each man knowing the affliction of his own heart."*** This is because in this world, we all go through diverse kinds of situations and temptations. And because our situations most times are so unique to us, no other person can truly understand what we are going through or feel our pain like we do. As the saying goes ***"He who wears the shoe knows where it pinches."***

If this is true, and it is, then it becomes inevitable that no one can truly pray for us with such fervor and intensity as we ourselves. After all, we are the ones with the pain and not the people we look up to for prayers. As ironic as it may sound, this same challenging life can be all fun for the man who has truly made prayer a lifestyle and is determined not to do anything without securing the help of God. By His superior wisdom and power, God has ordained our prayers to be a special avenue through which He will move in very special ways in our lives. And because no

One cherishes your priorities in life like you nor feel your pain like you,

You remain the best and the main man who can pray for you like no other. I truly believe that when a man is in partnership with his God on the altar of prayer, they become an unbeatable team.

Someone might reason, ***"But surely prayer can't make much difference. After all, if God in His sovereign will has already foreordained what is going to happen anyway-why even bother to pray?"*** A proper response is this: God sees every situation. He knew (in the past) if we would pray, and He worked our prayers into His plans. God (in His foreknowledge) has taken our prayers into consideration. True-we don't understand fully all that is involved, but we have been instructed and encouraged to pray-to pray about big things and little things, and to pray for our own needs as well as for the needs of others. I am thoroughly convinced that the Lord would never have put so much emphasis on praying, if indeed prayer had not been worthwhile. God's General, **Bob Gas,** rightly puts it this way, ***"if it's not big enough to be a prayer, then it's too small to be a burden,"***

We can be confident that prayer does change things because God worked our prayers into His plans, and though none of us can really

Explain it, but God has certain laws that only go into operation when

We sincerely pray! We must therefore begin to believe that God, in the mystery of prayer, has entrusted us with a force that can move the heavenly world, and can bring its power down to earth. I remember something beautiful that happened in one of our meetings 5 years ago. By then, I had been pastoring for two years and while ministering that Sunday morning on a message which I captioned ***"The word works",*** The lord impressed it upon my heart to pray for the supernatural move of his power so at the conclusion of the sermon, I took a bold step and said to the congregation that I have finished explaining the fact that the word of God works, now I want to prove it by praying for miracles to take place. On that note I asked that anyone in need of a miracle should step forward for the laying on of hands as we believed God for an instant testimony.

Friend, there was a sudden hush and unusual silence in church that morning as everyone looked on in amazement. They had never seen their pastor moving in the miraculous and so many wondered what I was up to that morning. Personally I was a bit calm and relaxed though I was giving such an invitation for the first time in my life. I was that

Relaxed because I was under the influence of the Holy Spirit and I was

Just taking a step of faith to do something unusual. But the doubt in the atmosphere was evident which almost intimidated me out of the place of faith. Suddenly, the silent atmosphere was interrupted positively as a certain pregnant lady walked to the platform in faith. When I asked her before the entire church what she wanted God to do for her, she said two things. First, she had carried the pregnancy to full term and the date the doctor gave her to be delivered of her baby had passed. Secondly, she didn't only want to put to birth, but she wants to be delivered of a baby girl. According to her, she had four boys already and the only reason she decided to have one more child is because she wanted to have a daughter amidst the boys, yet, her two times echography reveals that she's carrying another baby boy. So she wants me to pray and turn the sex of the baby.

Frankly speaking, the odds were beginning to weigh against my faith at her second request, coupled with the fact that another pregnant lady followed right after that request and came forward with a similar request even though she too was just a few weeks away from putting to birth. But you see, it's always a different set up when God ask you to

Do something and when you just choose to do it to feed your ego. My

Faith was up and it said yes to the challenge which made me believe God would not say NO.

So I laid my hands on her stomach and the moment I did, it was as though I touched a naked cable and some electrical waves ran through my hand. So I took my hands off immediately, then I turned to congregation and announced that the miracle has already taken place. The people clapped to encourage me in faith but then, I knew I wasn't just talking by faith but with a deep sense of knowing because of the signal I got so I went on to declare more words of protection and safe delivery. Then, as if to make matters worse, I now told her the baby will be born before the coming Sunday and that I will carry her daughter with my own hands before Sunday.

To the glory of God, my wife and I were out of town when my phone rang on Saturday morning by 10:00am as this dear lady was so pleased to call me by herself and deliver the news of her daughter's arrival. I immediately made the necessary arrangements and traveled back to town where we went to see her in the hospital and carried the baby that evening with our own hands, even as I said last year when we saw Princess Susan Ojong again after four years, she was already growi

Into a beautiful and lovely young lady. Truly, the thing that our God cannot do does not exist.

It is an error to think that the Christian life must really be a dull experience as some believe. They think and believe erroneously that to side with God is to terminate one's joy, pleasures and privileges. But the child of God has many wonderful privileges, and one of those privileges is access to God through the avenue of prayer. Think of it! We have the authority to come before the high and holy creator of the universe-and talk with Him! To have an audience (even once in a lifetime) with a king of a great nation (or the president of one's country) would be a special favor, and we would never forget it. But ours is an even greater privilege. We may have audience with the God who made us-not merely once in a lifetime, but day-in and day-out.

Certainly the avenue of prayer is a great privilege.

CHAPTER THREE

UNFORGETTABLE LEGACIES OF PRAYER

As children growing up in church, we were taught a lot of wonderful stories and truths in children's church. The influence my pastors and spiritual leaders had on me from childhood through different stages of growth was so strong. I couldn't have asked for a better foundation. I am whoever or whatever I am today because of the impact of the many wonderful men and women who gave their best to see me and many of my mates grow into responsible men and women. And I am glad, many of all those I grew up with are doing just fine in many aspects of their lives, especially in their spiritual lives.

As wonderful as the early knowledge of biblical truths were to me, one man that the teachings didn't particularly leave me with a good impression was the bible character called *Samson*. We were told that *Samson* was a powerful soldier but one who mingled with prostitutes and lived a very prayerless life. In fact, we were told that *Samson* prayed just once in his lifetime and that was on the day he was dying when he asked God to grant him the strength to pull down a gigantic building that ended up killing him and his tormentors. Actually,

Samson taking his revenge on his tormentors was one part of the story

I secretly admired because I myself was a very rough and very daring young man who would never let any mate of mine defeat me in a fight. If I had a fight with anybody and I was defeated, be rest assured the fight was not yet over. There had to be a second round of the encounter for which I will make sure I prepare so well that I will emerge the winner.

Back in 2015 when I officially began preaching, I preached with so much passion on a diverse number of subject yet, one of my most favorite and outstanding sermons was on the story of **Samson** and how dangerous it can be to live a prayerless life. And that the grace of God is always available to anyone at any point if only we will repent and return to God in prayers, even on our dying day. I made the point that it is never really over until it is all over, and it can only be all over when God makes his final statement, and that statement can be influenced by our prayers. I have held onto this notion that **Samson** never prayed one day in his whole life until recently as I was studying the amplified version of the Bible when the real facts were actually magnified before my very eyes. Please take a look at this passage.

And when he came to Lehi, the Philistines came shouting to meet him. And the spirit of the Lord came mightily upon [Samson], and the ropes on his arms became as flax that had caught fire, and his bonds melted off his hands. And he found a still moist jawbone of a donkey and reached out and took it and slew 1,000 men with it. And Samson said, with the jawbone of a donkey, heaps upon heaps, with the jawbone of a donkey I have slain 1,000 men! And when he stopped speaking, he cast the jawbone from his hand; and that place was called Ramath-lehi [the hill of the jawbone]. Samson was very thirsty, and he prayed to the Lord and said, you have given this great deliverance by the hand of your servant, and now shall I die of thirst and fall into the hands of the uncircumcised? And God split open the hollow place that was at Lehi, and water came out of it. And when he drank, his spirit returned and he revived. Therefore, the name of it was called En-hakkore [the spring of him who prayed], which is at Lehi to this day. And Samson judged (defended) Israel in the days of the Philistines twenty years. (Judges 15:14-20, Amp)

As you can see for yourself, ***Samson*** was a man who knew what it meant to pray and receive instant answers and manifestations from God. Samson was a man who left many great marks in Israel by the sheer force of his prayers. As a man who was surrounded by enemies seeking for his life time and again, I guess ***Samson*** understood what it meant to rely totally on God more than many of us do today. As the popular saying goes, ***"You will never know that God is all you need until God is all you've got."*** And all these things happened twenty years before the death of ***Samson*** as the scripture reveals.

Samson, in many occasions, as we have just read found himself suddenly in the midst of deadly enemies and problems he never saw coming but rose up boldly to the occasion because he was a man with a strong faith in God. You know, weak people pray to be kept out of unexpected problems while tough people pray for the strength to confront and conquer them. Life is full of many tough calls and unforeseen circumstances, but *Samson's* legacy shows us that what we need at such moments is not sympathy but strength. As a great man of God once said, ***"Victory is just a prayer away."***

GAINING MASTERY OF THE BATTLEFIELD

The story of ***Samson's "only but famous"*** prayer is told in ***Judges 16:1-30,*** wherein after the entire narrative of ***Samson's*** betrayal and torture, we read;

And when their hearts were merry, they said, call for Samson, that he may make sport for us. So they called [blind] Samson out of the prison, and he made sport before them. They made him stand between the pillars. And Samson said to the lad who held him by the hand, allow me to feel the pillars upon which the house rests, that I may lean against them. Now the house was full of men and women: all the philistine princes were there, and on the roof were about 3,000 men and women who looked on while Samson made sport. Then Samson called to the Lord and said, O Lord God [earnestly] remember me, I pray you, and strengthen me, I pray you, only this once, o God, and let me have one vengeance upon the Philistines for both my eyes. And Samson laid hold of the two middle pillars by which the house was borne up, one with his right hand and the other with his left. And Samson cried, let me die with the Philistines! And he bowed himself mightily, and the house fell upon the princes and upon all the people

That were in it. So the dead whom he slew at his death were more than they whom he slew in his life. (Judges 16:25-30, Amp)

Interesting!! Looking at the magnitude of ***Samson's*** accomplishments here, even logically looking at it, a man who has never practiced the art of prayer his whole life will not suddenly develop enough faith to begin praying for mighty miracles on a sick bed he landed on due to a crippling chronic sickness which is a similar description to what was happening here. I mean, if ***Samson*** had not experienced time and again what it means for God to answer prayers-both instantly and in time-he won't have had enough faith in God to pray that day for the first time in his life and believe God to execute such a mighty feat on the spot. Trying to convince me otherwise is like trying to tell me that a two- year-old boy once won a battle against a German military squad.

But you see, we can only become so good in the art of prayer and see mega results with time if we have been in the practice of it for some time. It's just like the significance of a story I came across many years

Ago about a Great War veteran who knew how to fight, not only in the physical but also by the spirit. According to a story circulated during World War I, a British soldier was caught one night while creeping secretively back to his tent from a nearby wooded area. He was immediately hauled before his commanding officer and charged with holding communications with the enemy. The man pleaded that he had gone into the woods to pray. That was his only defense.

"Have you been in the habit of spending hours in private prayer?" his officer asked roughly. *"Yes sir" "Then get down on your knees and pray now like you've never prayed before!"* the commander ordered. The young man knew he could be shot at sunrise for

the crime he was accused of committing. He knelt down and poured out his soul in a powerful prayer that could have only been inspired by the Holy Spirit. There was hushed silence after the soldier's amen.

"You may go," the officer finally said in hushed tones *"I believe your story. If you hadn't drilled often, you couldn't have done so well at review."*

I believe the commander's last statement explains my point so very clearly. The young soldier, on his part, didn't only pray always, but his prayers were effectual and fervent-they literally saved his life. He had a gun but didn't depend on it to see him through the war, he depended on the God he knew created him to keep him safe for the purpose he created him. The Psalmist said;

Some trust in chariots, and some in horses: but we will remember the name of the LORD our God.

(Ps

So from our little discussion about **Samson,** I believe it is evident enough for me to conclude that when

Samson prayed and said, **"...I pray you, only this**

once, O God…", he wasn't crying out of despair and saying O God answer me at least for once in my life. After all, he couldn't be expecting God to answer him a second time if he were only praying for the first time. What *Samson* was saying in essence was something like this, *"O God, I have had a very close and personal relationship with you all my life. And as a result, I have known what it means to be empowered by the spirit to the point where I*

Commanded the supernatural naturally. It is regrettable that my weakness and shortcomings in life have landed me in the hands of my enemies and made my end very miserable. I hereby accept the fact that my end is around the corner, but even if I have to die today, O God, you who has been in the habit of always answering my prayers, please answer me one more time and grant me the strength to terminate all these people who seek to destroy me. And God did! Which made the event another outstanding prayer legacy in Samson's profile.

THE PRAYER LEGACY OF JABEZ

In the book of Frist Chronicles, the Bible tells us about a man named Jabez. The first nine chapters consists of genealogies, listing more than six hundred names. And right there in the middle of all those names, God singles out one man for special recognition, and his name is Jabez. There are only two verses in the Bible about this man, yet he's given honorable mention above the six hundred other people mentioned in all those chapters.

Why did God single him out? What did Jabez do that caused his name?

To be preserved for over four thousand years? What made him above?

Average? What made God to give a distinguished testimony about Jabez?

"Now Jabez was more honorable than his brothers"

1 chronicles 4:9

So what set him apart? He dared to ask and believed God for great things. Let's look into the scriptures for a moment.

And Jabez was more honorable than his brethren: and his mother called his name Jabez, saying, Because I bare him with sorrow and Jabez called on God of Israel, saying, oh that thou wildest bless me indeed, and enlarge my coast, and that thine hand might be with me, and that thou wildest keep me from evil, that it may not grieve me! And God granted him that which he requested. (1 Chronicles 4:9-10, kjv)

The name Jabez means *"sorrow maker"* and as we very well know, a man's name is a pointer to his destiny. *Jabez's* mother named him sorrow maker because according to her testimony, she bore him in pain which provoked her to condemn his destiny. And according to the title

"Sorrow maker", the implication is that even if people and

Circumstances happen to play out in *Jabez's* favor at any point in time to give him peace and prosperity, somehow sorrow will be manufactured from nowhere to replace his joy because his identity was not synonymous with rest or laughter.

However, when *Jabez* grew up, he understood that though his mother had something to say about his life, he personally had much also to say about his destiny, which he did, and turned the tides around. Like **Jabez,** God wants us to be bold and daring when requesting things from him because it always takes a lionheart to secure a lion share. God wants us to ask Him for great things.

Jabez prayed that God would bless him in three specific ways:

1)   ***"Enlarge my coast."*** He had a dream of owning more land, and he asked God to bless that dream. It was a valid dream for ***Jabez*** and it is still a valid dream for us today. Reading through your bible, have you ever wondered why anytime God made promises to his children, he never fails to promise them their own land, amongst other things? I guess it's because God Almighty understands how important it is for every one of us to own his or her own piece of land. After all, land can

Only appreciate in value over time thereby making its owners wealthier by a huge margin. A life full of dreams is a life full of rich possibilities. When you stop dreaming you lose direction. When you stop setting goals you stop growing. You must have something you're pushing toward. As long as your horizon is expanding, you'll be spiritually and emotionally healthy.

2)   ***"That your hand would be with me."*** I love the content of ***Jabez's*** prayer because he asked for the best of things any man could possibly think of. He must have thought about his request carefully over an extended period of time before opening his mouth to make his request. God's hand here represents God's

power. ***Jabez*** realized that if he got more territory it meant he would have more responsibility, he would have greater demands and more pressure, and he would really need God's help in his life. So he requested God to be with him. And when you ask for God's presence in your life, you can be sure He'll answer.

3)   ***"That you would keep me from evil, that it may not grieve me"*** Finally, ***Jabez*** believing his new status will soon manifest was proactive and asked God for His protection. Why was this important?

Because in those days the more land you owned, the more influence you had, and the better known you were. And that made you a bigger target. It's still like that today. The more successful you are, the more critics you have. The more territory you own, the more your enemies will attack you. The closer you grow to the Lord and the stronger you become as a Christian, the more the devil will harass you because he doesn't want you to grow. But you can be sure, as ***Jabez*** was, that with God's protection you don't have to fear anyone or anything. Do you want to break out of mediocrity and human limitation? Then follow the example of ***Jabez.***

WHAT WILL YOUR LEGACY BE?

Jabez's brief but powerful story is a great inspiration and legacy to me. Not only did ***Jabez*** have great ambition, he had a growing faith and a deep trust in God. He had enough faith to pray and expect an answer. He was like the pioneer missionary ***William Carey***, who said, ***"Expect great things from God, and attempt great things for God."*** There's no mention of ***Jabez*** having any special ability or talent. The Bible doesn't say he was wealthy or educated. He was simply a common man with an uncommon faith. Don't worry about what you don't have-if you

Have faith! God is in the business of honoring people's faith and He will give you the necessary power. It gives God so much pleasure to use ordinary people who are willing to trust Him, and see them succeed. Lots of super-talented people sit on the sidelines while ordinary people with faith score the goals and win. And you can be one of them.

THINK ON THESE THINGS

"A man who knows what is good for him does not wait until the last minute before doing it."

-Tabot Henry Ojo

CHAPTER FOUR

FIRST THINGS FIRST

After all is and said done, friend, if you really want to see the hand of God on your life, not only in this world, but to also prepare and keep you for the good life that can only be found in his bosom in the great beyond, then you need to start by acknowledging Jesus Christ, the Son of the one and only true living God, as your personal Lord and Savior.

Therefore, if you are not yet a believer in and follower of God, please you need to start now by taking this simple confession of faith. With an open and expectant heart, please open your mouth and repeat this prayer after me;

DEAR LORD JESUS. TODAY I HAVE RECEIVED YOUR WORD AND I ACKNOWLEDGE THAT IT WAS WRITTEN FOR ME. THEREFORE I BELIEVE IN THE WORDS I HAVE RECEIVED. I ACKNOWLEDGE THAT I AM A SINNER OH GOD. I CONFESS AND FORSAKE ALL MY SINS NOW. I INVITE YOU DEAR LORD JESUS TO COME INTO MY LIFE NOW AND TAKE OVER MY ENTIRE BEING AND PERSONALITY. I CONFESS WITH MY OWN MOUTH THAT I AM NOW BORN AGAIN. I BELIEVE I HAVE RECEIVED SALVATION FOR MY SOUL NOW AND I AM A CHILD OF GOD NOW AND FOREVER. SO HELP ME DEAR LORD TO LIVE FOR YOUR GLORY NOW AND

FOREVER AMEN.

If you prayed that prayer with me, I want to welcome you into God's family and I want to assure you that this is the best decision you could ever take for your life. Now that you're born again, I pray that the hand of God will be strong on your life and that God will do for you what He has been doing for all his other children. I declare your sins forgiven now, therefore receive the peace of God for your mind and receive the gift of the Holy Spirit for the manifestation of a new you. Go forth now and show the world what it means to be blessed IN JESUS MIGHTY NAME! AMEN.

I also encouraged you to get to a good study Bible for yourself, join a Bible believing church and be committed to the teachings and leadership of the Holy

Spirit for your new life in Christ. No man ever serves God and regrets it. No one becomes committed to God and ends a loser in life.it pays to serve God! He's not known for doing try by error with people's lives, he won't begin with you. God is not a user but a blesser of men. You will not seek him in vain. Once more, congratulations for your new found life in Christ Jesus. You're blessed for life!!